Essential Oils- The Ultimate Resource

A Beginner's Guide to the Use of Essential Oils

By: Amy Zulpa

TABLE OF CONTENTS

PUBLISHERS NOTES

Disclaimer

This publication is intended to provide helpful and informative material. It is not intended to diagnose, treat, cure, or prevent any health problem or condition, nor is intended to replace the advice of a physician. No action should be taken solely on the contents of this book. Always consult your physician or qualified health-care professional on any matters regarding your health and before adopting any suggestions in this book or drawing inferences from it.

The author and publisher specifically disclaim all responsibility for any liability, loss or risk, personal or otherwise, which is incurred as a consequence, directly or indirectly, from the use or application of any contents of this book.

Any and all product names referenced within this book are the trademarks of their respective owners. None of these owners have sponsored, authorized, endorsed, or approved this book.

Always read all information provided by the manufacturers' product labels before using their products. The author and publisher are not responsible for claims made by manufacturers.

Manufactured in the United States of America

DEDICATION

This book is dedicated to my dear friend Melissa who introduced me to the wonderful world of essential oils.

Chapter 1- What Are Essential Oils?

Just imagine: It's a beautiful day outside. You are running in a park surrounded by gorgeous trees and flowers. If you think a little deeper, you realize that you are surrounded by all kinds of essential oils.

Essential oils are extracted from flowers, leaves, tree bark, seeds, berries, roots, stems, fruits or twigs. Essential oils are highly concentrated potent liquids that do not feel oily. Other names of essential oils are aromatherapy oils, volatile oils, ethereal oils or aetherolea. Our ancestors started to use the oils hundreds if not thousands of years ago because they discovered the therapeutic effects the oils can have.

One of the ways to use these oils is to rub them on skin. Before you start actively using essential oils do an allergy test. Rub a small area of skin with some diluted oil. Look for skin redness or other painful reactions. Be ready, you can experience irritation. If that happens, do not use that oil. However, the majority of people use essential oils without having any allergic reactions.

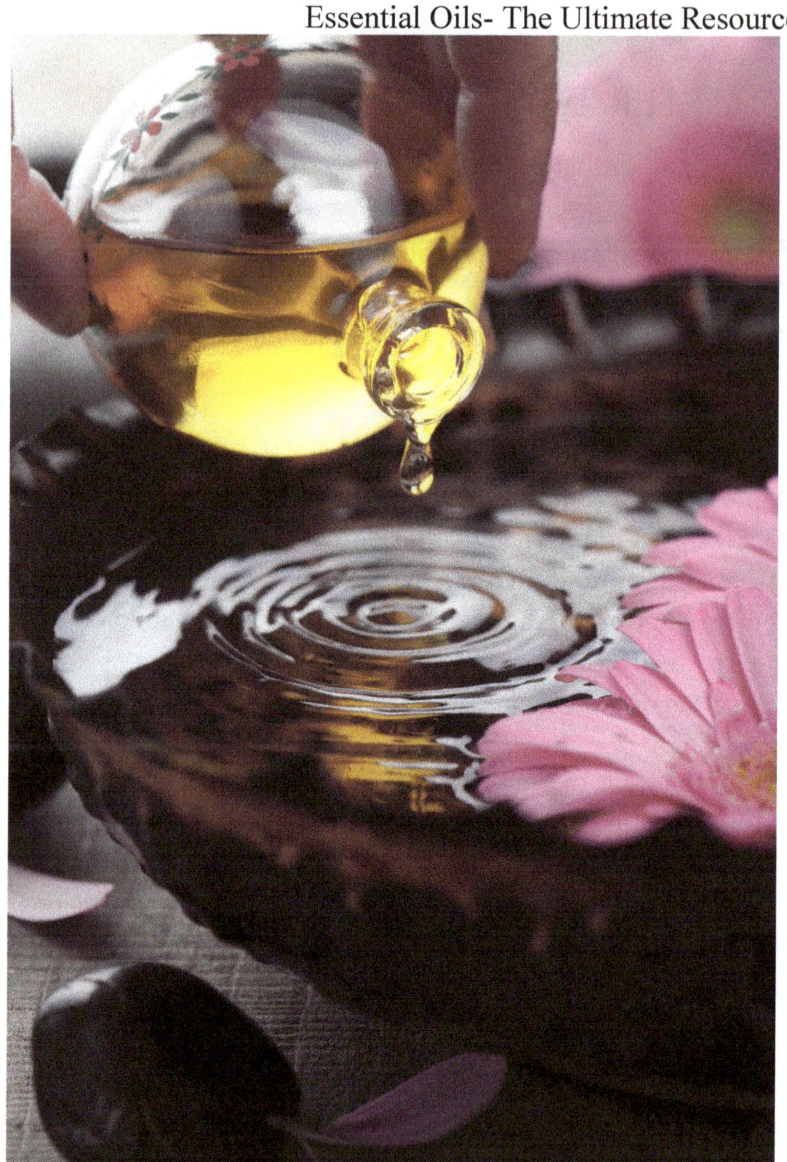

Is My Oil Fake Or Real?

Essential oils are very popular. Maybe this is the reason for a lot of misinformation about the oils. Have you ever heard about "essential oils party"? People sell oils everywhere: on eBay, Etsy and through local newspapers, just to name a few. Some people try to sell pure oils at very low prices. Some body and bath products claim to use pure essential oils that do not exist. Plumeria is one of them. Know this fact: it takes 150 pounds of raw lavender to make one pound of lavender oil.

Let's talk about genuine rose oil. Pure natural rose oil is very expensive. It takes 200 pounds or 60,000 rose flowers to make one ounce of rose oil. If you bought a five milliliter bottle of rose oil and paid less than $80, there is something wrong. It could be synthetic oil. It also could be natural diluted oil. Please, use common sense when you buy essential oils.

The persons that sell these oils can make genuine mistakes. You need to know the true reputation of who you are buying the oils from. If you buy oils with the wrong labels, you open yourself to possible allergies, skin sensitivity, irritations and skin outbreaks. Bear in mind that there are no standard official regulations that govern usage of essential oils.

How to Use Peppermint Oil

Peppermint oil can be used as a mouth freshener. If you just had coffee, salsa or something that had garlic in it, you might want to refresh your breath. Peppermint oil is perfect for that. Dip a toothpick into a bottle with peppermint oil and mix pure water with it. You will make a perfectly healthy water rinse that will stay with you for quite some time. Rinse your mouth and gargle. Did you know that most oils kill bacteria and prevent gum disease?

Peppermint oil can also be used to relieve dizziness or headache. Rub a drop or two of peppermint oil slowly on your temples. Use circular motions. It will give you pleasant cooling effect and relieve the pain.

How to Improve Your Mood by Using a Mix of Lavender and Rose Oils

Lavender oil works great when mixed with rose oil. Use the mixture in a diffuser. The scent will spread out. In about 30 to 60 minutes you will start feeling relaxed and calm.

How to Use Bergamot Oil to Beautify Your Skin

Skin is the largest organ of the human body. It's not easy to keep your skin perfect. Bergamot oil will help fight these skin problems: acne, eczema, cold sores, psoriasis, dark spots and dull & dry complexion. It will also help you to relieve anxiety and stress.

Bergamot oil is made from bergamot fruit peel. Bergamot fruit is an orange that looks like a pear! The scientific name of it is "citrus bergamia". The peel has the color of a lemon and it grows naturally in Lombardy, Italy. Bergamot can be used to make some fantastic marmalade.

Adding bergamot to your skin care formula will help keep it clear of acne because bergamot makes your skin resistant to microorganisms. Bergamot kills facial bacteria before your skin creates blackheads and pimples. It also controls excess oil production in the skin. If you decide to use bergamot for as a skin care product, you will not need to use chemically based cleansing products.

Bergamot oil fosters healing of the skin and also helps it to regenerate. Do you have old acne scars, psoriasis, cold sores, skin scars, stretch marks or eczema? Bergamot oil will help your skin to heal faster. Bergamot can also be combined with other oils to help with other ailments.

These Essential Oils Encourage Hair Growth

Lavender Oil

Chamomile Oil

Rosemary

Peppermint

Lemon

Myrrh

Some distributors claim that essential oils bring nutrients to your body. Robert Tisserand, aromatherapist and the author of "The Art of Aromatherapy" (Healing Arts Press, 1978), mentioned in his book that essential oils do not contain nutrients, minerals, vitamins, amino acids, proteins, carbohydrates, or any other type of nutrient. Note however that essential oils cannot cure cancer or any other diseases.

Keep in mind, the information you read in this book is not intended to diagnose or cure diseases. Use common sense and advice of a medical doctor if you have a health problem.

Chapter 2- What Are the Intrinsic Benefits of Using Essential Oils?

As mentioned in chapter one, there are many different kinds or types of essential oils. Each kind of essential oil is beneficial and helpful to your health in some way or other.

One type of essential oil is peppermint. The benefits of peppermint go way beyond refreshing your breath. It can assist with stomach issues such as indigestion and queasiness. It can also stop itching and help with muscles that are hurting you. You can add some droplets of essential oil to a bowl of scalding water and then breathe in the steam. This oil should help clear a stuffy nose. You could also rub the peppermint water into your muscles that are sore. If you are a woman, it can help you to relieve menstrual cramps. Sore throats and head pain can be soothed with peppermint. It can be a replacement for caffeine.

The next essential oil to look at is lavender. The main benefit of lavender essential oil appears to be its antibacterial attributes. It has had great success at fighting germs in the home as well as the body. It can also fight indigestion as well as head pain, just like peppermint.

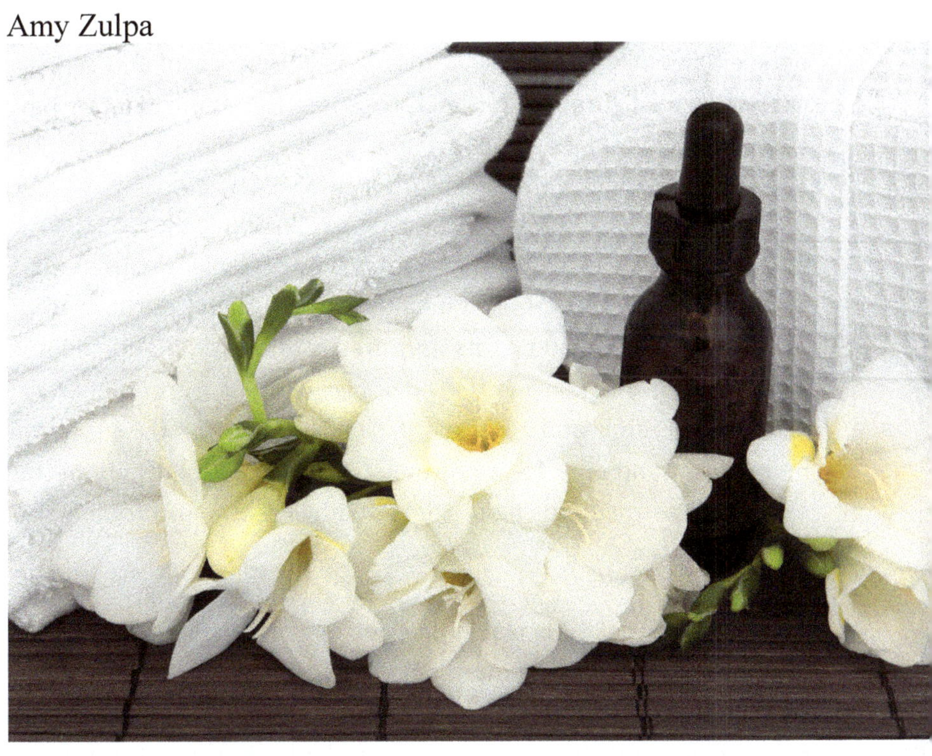

The smell of lavender can calm you, make sleep better, help relieve the pain in your joints and help you with urinary ailments, heart problems, pimples and high blood pressure.

The next essential oil that can be examined is sesame. It is considered a critical component of hair and skin treatment, due to its hydrating attributes.

It has other benefits. It can adequately protect you from the sun with its slight sun protection factor. It has adequate fatty acids to decrease stress, lower blood pressure and slow the growth of cancer in cells.

The benefits of geranium can be looked at next. It can also be mixed with other oils to help alleviate menstrual cramps. It helps to rejuvenate the skin by stopping the inflammations and hemorrhages in the skin. It has had remarkable success in treating pimples and oily skin as well. It is able to get rid of the scarring caused by disfigurements and blemishes. Geranium oil can have you looking younger as over time it does help to reduce the appearance of lines and wrinkles that come with age.

Pine is not only a smell that reminds everyone Christmas; it is another essential oil. Holistic health experts would put it on their top ten lists as a result of its germfree, antibacterial and sedative attributes. It has success in helping with skin problems like psoriasis, eczema and pimples. It can also help to speed up the metabolism and cure food poisoning, make your joint pain better, eliminate germs and help those with breathing problems to breathe better.

Another essential oil is clove, particularly spicy clove oil. This spicy oil is a part of the components in Tiger Balm. Tiger Balm is supposed to be a remedy to do away with your hangover head pain. Holistic health people are able to find other uses for it. If you have dental issues like teeth and gum pain, you should use this oil Clove oil can also help the keep the breath fresh.

Another benefit of spicy clove oil is that it is good at treating bug bites, cuts and scrapes. The oil can also be used in the ear, stomach, nose and head.

Your sex life might be improved as it is said to help with the libido.

There are certain dos and don’ts to using essential oils. You should never apply an essential oil directly to your skin. You should dilute it first.

The best way to apply essential oils to your body is by taking a bath. You should add eight to ten droplets of essential oil to the water and then get in, lean back and relax. Jasmine, Roman chamomile, frankincense, lavender and grapefruit are the recommended essential oils to put in bath water.

After you do a workout, you should use eucalyptus essential oil to soothe your aches and pains in your muscles and joints.

Another effective way to use essential oils is to breathe it in. It will have a positive effect on your mood. Breathing in essential oils can help to put the mind at ease. You should add five to ten droplets of oil to steaming water. This water should not be boiling. You then put a towel over your head. You should breathe in deeply and repeat the process. You will be surprised at the positive effect this has on the body and the nasal passages as well.

You can also try putting some droplets of your favorite essential oil on your pillow before going to sleep. It will help you to relax and sleep through the night.

To take things a step further you can buy a humidifier and add five to ten droplets of essential oil to the humidifier twice a day.

Another good way to apply essential oil is by compaction. You should compact for relaxation, head pain, menstrual pain, sore muscles and many other body problems. You should add five to ten droplets of essential oil (usually peppermint) to a tiny bowl of scalding water. You should dip a towel in, get rid of excess water and press to the ailing area. You should repeat the process until the towel cools.

You can also aerate the home with essential oils. The oils can naturally purge the air. You can spread the pleasant odor of essential oils by heating or burning the essential oil.

You can also put your favorite essential oils in spray bottles. You use them to spray the oils on clothes, bed sheets and rugs. You could also spray them throughout the house. Essential oils help to get rid of fungus, germs, dust mites and bad odors. You could have one bottle with Roman Chamomile to help calm things down at bedtime and one bottle containing frankincense for the morning time.

Chapter 3- How to Use Essential Oils Safely- Purchasing, Storing and Blending

Essential oils have been used throughout history to cure all many ailments that plague mankind. Used topically, or, in some cases, internally, essential oils are powerful tools that can be used to help bring about natural healing in countless situations. In recent years, with the climbing cost associated with traditional health care, more and more people are looking to essential oils to help themselves and their loved ones live healthier happier lives. However, the use of essential oils is not something that should be taken lightly. For anyone looking to collect study and use essential oils, there are some important aspects to consider.

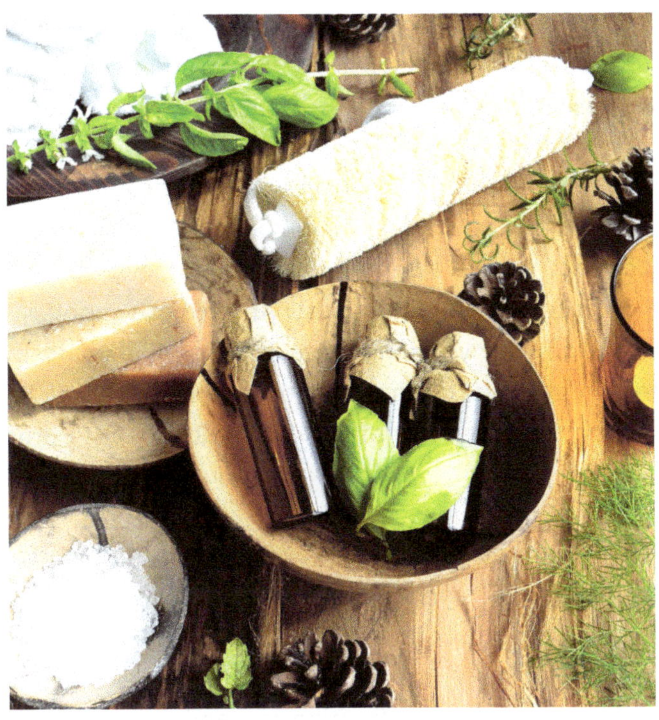

Perhaps the most obvious question many beginners have is where to purchase essential oils. Chances are you will not find them on the self at your local grocery store stocked next to the vegetable oil and cooking spray. There are many outlets available to purchase your essential oils from. With the wide spread access to the Internet that many have these days, the easiest way for most people will likely be to shop for essential oils online. Health food stores maybe also carry a selection of essential oils for you to choose from.

Locating your nearest health food store is a great start to finding the essential oils you want to work with. Also, you may want to check out nearby country pharmacies, as they sometimes carry a mix of new medicine as well as medicine from a simpler time. Being able to go to a store near you is the best way to be sure that what you are getting is what you want. Shopping this way also helps you make doubly sure that you are getting fresh product as stores rotate their inventory. On top of that, there is the added bonus of being able to ask the person running the store questions about your purchase in case you need assistance.

While shopping locally for your oil is highly recommended, there can be problems. For starters, finding a local health food store or pharmacy that carries essential oils may not even be an option simply because one does not exist. And, what's more, if you do have a physical store you can peruse, you may find yourself looking for a certain essential oil that they do not have in stock or simply do not carry and you may not be able to get them to order it for you.

Thankfully, if you have an Internet connection, the world is your oyster. There are a number of reputable outlets where you can purchase your essential oils and have them shipped directly to you. These online stores are usually able to offer you a bigger selection of oils than any one physical location can, and at a lower price.

Some of the downsides to purchasing your essential oils online are that you are buying them sight unseen. The seller could be selling some diluted form of the oil without telling you, or even selling you older product that is no longer fit for use. Make sure that you always buy from places with good reviews and sterling reputations before you buy.

Any type of natural oil can go bad if stored improperly. Essential oils are no different. The first thing to always look for is that the oils are in amber glass bottles. Amber glass bottles help protect the oils in two ways. Direct light will degrade the integrity of the oil. The amber tint is more effective at reducing the amount of light that passing through the bottle than clear or green tinted glass. The fact that the bottle is made of glass is also important as it is not made with synthetic materials that could damage your oils the way a plastic container might. Make sure you store your oils in a cool, dry place out of direct sunlight and they should keep practically forever.

The blending of essential oils is extremely important, not only to address your specific need, but also to ensure that the oils used do not cause harm to the user. Essential oils are also known as volatile oils because in their pure, undiluted form, they can actually burn the skin when used topically or make someone very ill when they are ingested. It is necessary that you mix your essential oils with “carrier" oil in order to dilute it. The general rule is to aim for a 2-2.5% dilution for adults and 1% for children. A good way to make sure you dilute your essential oil enough is to add 1 drop of essential oil to a every teaspoon of carrier oil. You can use cold pressed olive oil or coconut oil to accomplish this, or even add the essential oil to lotions, shampoos or mouthwash, depending on how you use it.

Essential oils can be an awesome ally in your fight to stay healthy and keep medical expenses to a minimum. While these potent oils are nothing to be toyed with, with some adequate reading and a healthy dose of caution, you can learn how to harness their power and improve your quality of life. As long as you remember to always buy from reputable shops, whether they are bought locally or online, to store your oils in a dark, cool, dry area in amber glass bottles, and to blend them with other oils in order to make them safe for use, there are no limits to what you will be able to heal.

CHAPTER 4- WHICH ESSENTIAL OILS HELP CARE FOR THE SKIN?

Have you ever walked by the skin care aisle of a health food store and wondered about all those mysterious bottles of essential oils? You may be curious about some essential oils that have been around for thousands of years (remember frankincense and myrrh from the Bible?). Navigating the world of natural skin care can be intimidating, but the following is an introductory guide to which essential oils can help with skin health. Taking the first step to understanding how essential oils can be beneficial for the skin can be an exciting foray into a more holistic approach to life.

As mentioned through this book, there are different ways that essential oils can be absorbed into the body: through ingestion, inhalation, and topical skin application. This chapter will only discuss the essential oils that can be applied to the skin. Essential oils may be applied to the skin by massage, using compresses, sprays, or baths.

It is a good idea to purchase essential oils that are 100% pure and natural in order for them to be most effective and beneficial. Because essential oils are so concentrated, most essential oils need to be diluted with a carrier oil, such as olive oil, sweet almond oil, grape seed oil, avocado oil, sunflower oil, or jojoba oil. Follow the directions on the essential oils bottle when deciding if and how dilution should occur.

A word of caution on natural skin care--using pure, natural, and chemical-free essential oils does not necessarily mean you don't need to be cautious about how you apply the essential oils. Even though a product may be natural, you may still be sensitive or allergic to it. Essential oils are generally quite potent so irritation may occur if not used correctly. If you are trying an essential oil for the first time, it is a good idea to test it out first by applying a small amount on the inside of your upper arm. Wait a few hours and see if any redness or itching develops. Doing a little research on the internet, referencing aromatherapy books or a consultation with an aromatherapist can minimize any problems from essential oil usage.

This introductory guide to essential oils for skin care does not cover a comprehensive list of skin ailments that can be addressed with essential oils. Rather, here is a list of essential oils that have been found to be suitable for most skin types and can be a good start to incorporate into your skin care regimen.

Geranium Essential Oil: This is a multi-purpose essential oil that is ideal for all skin types. It can address skin issues such as healing wounds, fading scars and spots. It is said to promote cell growth as well. Geranium essential oil should be diluted before application to the skin.

Rose Essential Oil: Rose essential oil is more expensive and difficult to find but it has numerous uses. Rose essential oil is said to be effective for dry and aging skin. It also has astringent properties that helps with thread veins/broken capillaries. Furthermore, rose essential oil can also help fade scars, acne marks and stretch marks (said to be ideal during pregnancy but consult a doctor if concerned about safety). There are two types of rose essential oils: rose otto and rose absolute. Rose otto is the more superior grade.

Rosehip Essential Oil: This essential oil contains Omega 3,6 and 9, vitamin C, lycopene and linoleum acids, which help with moisturizing the skin, regenerating skin cells, minimizing the signs of aging, reducing fine lines, and boosting collagen. This oil is considered to be one of the predominant oils used for treating wrinkles and premature aging. This oil is more gentle so it may be used undiluted on the skin if desired.

Tea Tree Oil: This versatile essential oil is best suited for oily or acne prone skin. Additionally, it is possibly effective for medicinal purposes, such as treating warts, athlete's foot, bug bites, fungal infections, abrasions, and cold sores. This oil is potent so be more cautious when using it.

Bergamot Essential Oil: Bergamot essential oil is also better suited for oily or acne prone skin. Its antiviral properties can help fight off cold sores as well as help reduce oil, acne and bacteria on your skin.

Sandalwood Essential Oil: Sandalwood essential oil is beneficial for your skin and hair. It is suitable for most skin types, but is particularly helpful for cracked and chapped skin. It may be effective in reducing lines, healing and reducing scars and reviving tired, dull skin. You can also use this oil on your hair to increase moisture levels and shine.

There are many ways to use essential oils, so it may be fun for you to experiment a little. Just to give you a few ideas, essential oils can be added to your facial cleansers, you can make your own serums, or you can do a quick facial steam. Besides being beneficial for the skin, many essential oils have other health benefits (i.e. calming and elevating one's mood).

It's important to remember that essential oils are very concentrated, so a little goes a long way. As you start experimenting with different oils you may find some work better for you than others. There are many other beneficial essential oils that have not been discussed in this chapter, but the short list above can be good essential oils to start with if you are interested in incorporating natural skin care products into your life.

Chapter 5- Which Essential Oils Help Heal the Body?

Many consumers today want to return to homeopathic remedies that utilize natural resources to maintain their overall health. This trend stems from a number of different sources. For example, common side effects that could result from taking prescription medications are often much worse than the underlying condition they are designed to treat in the first place. Another reason for the preference of natural remedies is the idea that adding manmade chemicals and byproducts to the body can cause unwanted and irreversible changes to the physiology. People are more educated and aware of how easily the brain and body can become addicted to chemical substances, processed foods and learned behavior.

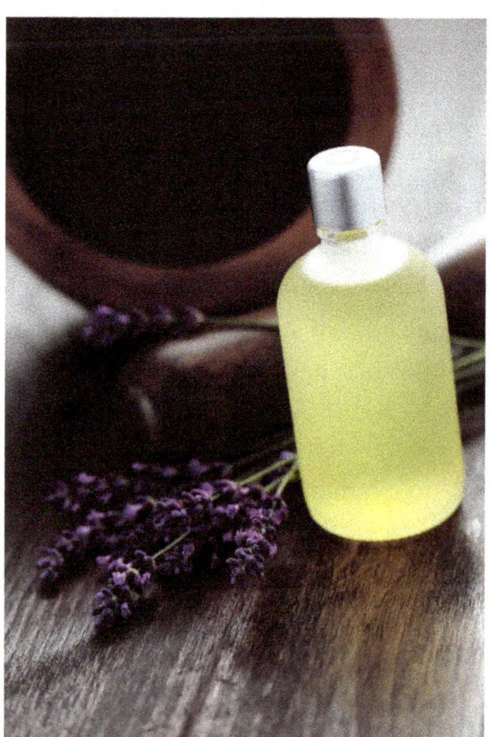

Ancient Customs

Most every ancient civilization used oils for a variety of purposes. Some of these uses were based on religious or spiritual beliefs, such as anointing or embalming bodies before burial, while others were later proven to be at least somewhat sound and scientifically based. Following the patterns of established ancient customs has been successful in treating a myriad of ailments and diseases that occur in the modern world. Many of these sacred treatments involve the use and application of essential oils.

Tea Tree Oil

This popular oil, extracted primarily from the Australian Melaleuca Alternifolia plant, has many practical uses for the home, as well as healing properties for various ailments. Tea tree oil is an effective treatment for blisters, minor abrasions, open wounds and acne because it produces a protective covering for new skin growth and it also provides medicinal compounds that counteract specific bacteria known to cause skin infections. It has also been used topically to treat pink eye and can be inhaled with steam or swallowed to relieve sore throat pain.

Lavender

The lavender flower is actually an herb, and certain species of this plant are used for an untold number of healing properties. The most popular commercial use of lavender is for aromatherapy and relaxation. This feature is marketed in many ways, from infant bath formulas to attention deficit disorders and even heating oil face wash and moisturizers for adults. Lavender has a wonderful aroma that acts as a natural decongestant, making it useful for treating allergies, asthma and the common cold. The oils from this herb are also useful for treating skin conditions such as blisters and burns.

Lavender is also used for opening clogged pores or tear ducts and even clearing up pink eye.

Thieves Oil

This blend of five separate essential oils has potent antibacterial and antiviral properties that are often used to fight various infections. The common cold, canker sores, mouth ulcers, chicken pox, herpes and other viruses are combated by the aromatic and powerful oil when applied or ingested. Thieves oil was created by combining the known effects of cloves, cinnamon bark, eucalyptus, lemon and rosemary into one essential oil that has the ability to diffuse airborne bacteria when sprayed or absorbed into the atmosphere. The specific blend is also useful to treat coughs and chest congestion, ear infections, sore throats, bronchitis and headaches.

Eucalyptus

Found as part of a blend in thieves' oil, eucalyptus has been used independently for centuries as a treatment for sinus congestion, and other chronic respiratory disorders. The flowering tree from Australia offers a wide range of healing properties other than being a decongestant. Eucalyptus offers anti-inflammatory and anti-spasmodic benefits for individuals suffering from chronic conditions. This pleasant aroma can be used as an effective antiseptic and also as a natural stimulant to fight off afternoon sleepiness or long-term fatigue. Aromatherapy blends that are designed to be inhaled or used in a steam room often contain Eucalyptus.

Sandalwood

Oils from the fragrant Sandalwood tree offer users a variety of health benefits, including stress reduction and aromatherapy.

Sandalwood has been used as a natural sedative for centuries to induce restful sleep and relax users. The rich oil is also helpful to treat dry, chapped skin and lips, as well as replenishing natural oils from the skin after serious sunburn, wind burn or other burns. Most recently, sandalwood oil has been used to reduce or eliminate symptoms of Alzheimer's disease and as a cancer prevention measure. Sandalwood stimulates the pineal gland, creating the relaxation and stress reduction qualities, and also helps in the treatment of depression and anxiety.

Frankincense

Also known as olibanum, frankincense is often used for making perfumes and incense. In ancient times, the oil from these trees was often given as a gift to new the parents of newborn babies because of its relaxation properties. Today, people use frankincense oil to help relax and counteract anxiety, stress, high blood pressure and other common ailments. It can be used as a body oil, deodorant, perfume or simply rubbed directly on the feet, wrists or hands to release its properties. Frankincense can also be applied topically to prevent or reduce symptoms of Alzheimer's disease.

Peppermint

Most oils from the mint family have aromatic properties that aid in healing problems associated with the respiratory system. The peppermint flower is actually a hybrid mixture of spearmint and water mint. Because it is readily available for harvest on nearly every continent, peppermint has been in constant demand for several centuries, with each generation adding new uses based on the versatile properties. More than any other essential oil, peppermint is highly recommended for treating disorders of the digestive system such as nausea, cramps and heartburn. It is also an effective treatment for nerve pain such as toothaches and headaches.

Chapter 6- Which Essential Oils Are Best For Massages?

For anyone who has ever gotten a massage, he or she knows how relaxing and wonderful they feel. There really isn't anything like the muscles in the body receiving a massage that is fit for a king. Of course, there are several benefits beyond the fact that massages feel good on the body. And while some are better than others, it is important to find a masseuse or masseur that is well crafted in the art. Likewise, the products that these professionals use matter, and there are essential massage oils that take the experience to a new level of gratification.

As a soothing massage will allow you much needed relaxation after a long day, it also provides other wonderful healthy benefits. Feel the oils being gently applied to your body to add a whole new level to the experience. Many of these oils that will bring a healthy feeling to you can make all the difference in how the massage goes with the various oils providing their own set of benefits. Whether you get an at-home massage from a loved one, or spend the big bucks hiring a professional, the best massage oils should be used. Breathe in deep and trust these products to get it done.

The very best massage oils are those that are made of natural products that are actually good for the skin. You simply don't want to use one that makes your skin break out in boils and hives, so it is important to know what is being used on your body. Using the wrong oils will counteract the wonderful healing benefits of a massage. The first massage oil that comes to mind is found in almonds. Yes, the super nut also provides healthy massage oils.

Other than those who are allergic to nuts, the oil extracted from almonds will not cause unhealthy reactions on the skin. Sweet almond oil may be a pale yellow color, but you'll feel marvelous when this oily texture is applied to your skin. This massage oil is widely used by many for a reason, as it allows the hands to move easily along the skin and isn't absorbed quickly, meaning it won't have to be applied every other minute to get that slick surface. Sweet almond oil is one of those essential oils that need to be used in a massage, unless of course the receiver s allergic to nuts. It is reasonably priced and works like a charm, but isn't the only oil to consider using with a massage.

Consider using jojoba oil extracted from the jojoba plant for a grand massage. We list it as oil, but technically it is a wax that comes from the seed of the plant. It is not only perfect to use during a full body massage, but it also is thought to have antibacterial properties that can clear acne-filled pores. Jojoba oil is preferred by many massage therapists for its ability to be well-absorbed, have a very long shelf life and the fact that it is unlikely to irritate the skin. Unlike sweet almond oil, however, jojoba oil has a tendency to be absorbed quickly, forcing you to reapply it quite often. But that is hardly a blemish on this wonderful massage oil.

You've heard of coconut oil being used in the kitchen, but it can also be effectively used on the massage table. When thinking of coconut oil, naturally one may picture something along the lines of a thick white paste. The coconut oil used for massages is called fractionated coconut oil and it is far less thick than that used in the kitchen, as it is only a fraction of that. This oil is light and non-greasy, a perfect combination. Like sweet almond oil, is relatively cheap, all while lasting a long time. It also won't stain, so you can use it on the massage bed and not worry about making a permanent stain in the sheets.

Apricot kernel oil is rich in Vitamin E, making it last long on your shelf. This oil will certainly be absorbed easily and the skin and won't make you feel like you've been rolling around in baby oil for hours, after your massage. Apricot kernel oil is essential massage oil for those who are unable to use a product that has a high concentration of nuts, such as the sweet almond oil, as it has very similar properties without disrupting the allergies.

Speaking of nut allergies, don't use the wonderful sunflower oil if you are allergic to the plant or nut. Otherwise, sunflower oil is a very good massage oil. It won't leave you feeling greasy afterwards. It has several properties in it that leave the skin happy and healthy, including palmitic and linoleic acid. Unlike all of the aforementioned essential massage oils, sunflower oil tends to go bad quickly. Keep this in mind when buying it, procuring the oil in small doses. Store it in a dark cool area when not using this terrific massage oil.

Everything needs to go right when it comes to the perfect massage. This includes the oils being used on the body when the rub down is taking place. And while a massage has plenty of healthy attributes associated with the practice, putting unhealthy oils on the skin during one, will be extremely counter-intuitive. Loosen up, use the right oils and let the massage take away muscle pain and anxiety. Massages are meant to inspire happy thoughts and to bring peace of mind.

Chapter 7- Which Essential Oils Help Keep the Hair Healthy?

Essential oils are centuries-old, organic, hair care stimulants. In this modern age, people use a variety of mineral/petroleum emollients and their many byproducts. Unfortunately, research proves that these are not the best options available to reach rewarding results. The hair needs nutrient-furnishing elements to stimulate growth naturally and receive full protection. Education is the key to use essential oils properly. As plant-based ingredients, it helps to know the usefulness of each element found in distilled essential oils. There's a rich blend of properties found in the extracts. Continue reading to learn the truth behind using natural essential oils to restore volume, strength and systematize defense in the hair.

Growth Enhancing, Moisture Replenishing, Scalp Cleansing Tea-Tree Oil

Known to offer a prolific range of health benefits, Tea tree oil is an unfailing hair treatment. It has a profuse source of ingredients that restores moisture to the hair evenly as it keeps the scalp bacteria-free. In addition, it stimulates the sebaceous glands to improve the flow of the scalp's biological moisturizer elements. In the process, it removes all dead skin cells to promote the growth of new ones. This puts a stop to the formation and progression of dandruff. Besides, the hair is likely to develop an inhospitable atmosphere to parasites and fungal infections. This owes to the biological anti-fungal, antibacterial agents found in this essential oil that constantly cleans and protects the follicles.

Myrrh Oil: Natural, Scalp-Healing Moisturizer

Myrrh Oil is another useful natural hair treatment. The extracted oil offers a rich blend of potent ingredients to treat dry, itchy scalp. In addition, it prevents and controls dandruff problems by giving the roots enough moisture. This all-natural essential oil formula works best to treat dry hair types.

Odor-Blocking, Strands Strengthening Lavender Oil

Lavender Oil has active properties that treat different hair and scalp conditions. It has a refreshing aroma that keeps the tresses smelling garden-fresh and healthy. As a treatment for all hair types, there's no limit to its potency. When distilled, this essential oil treats serious cases of hair loss, breakage and scalp itchiness. Additionally, it is a miracle-working growth formula to repair and strengthen damaged tresses. This regrowth formula is ideal to treat Alopecia and other stages of excessive baldness. There's no restriction on age and gender.

Scalp-Cleansing, Hair Repairing, Aromatic Rosemary Oil

The extracts of the Rosemary plant create aromatic blends of essential oils to treat the hair. Similar to Lavender EO, it keeps the hair refreshed and odor-free. Distilled rosemary oil is the perfect stimulant the hair needs to strengthen the roots. This is to stimulate the regrowth of stronger, longer tresses naturally. Besides, the antibacterial, stimulating substances it contains help to slow down dandruff progression. Essentially, it repairs and cleans the follicles to stop the cycle of excruciating, flaking, dry scalp conditions.

Deep-Cleansing, Hair-Restoring Chamomile Essential Oil

Known for its nerve-soothing effects on the body, chamomile oil works similar when used in the hair. This is approvingly a signature feature of this essential oil. Additionally, it is a safe, extremely efficacious hair care solution to remove inactive skin cells. This helps to develop a healthy atmosphere to stimulate the follicles to sprout thicker, longer strands of hair.

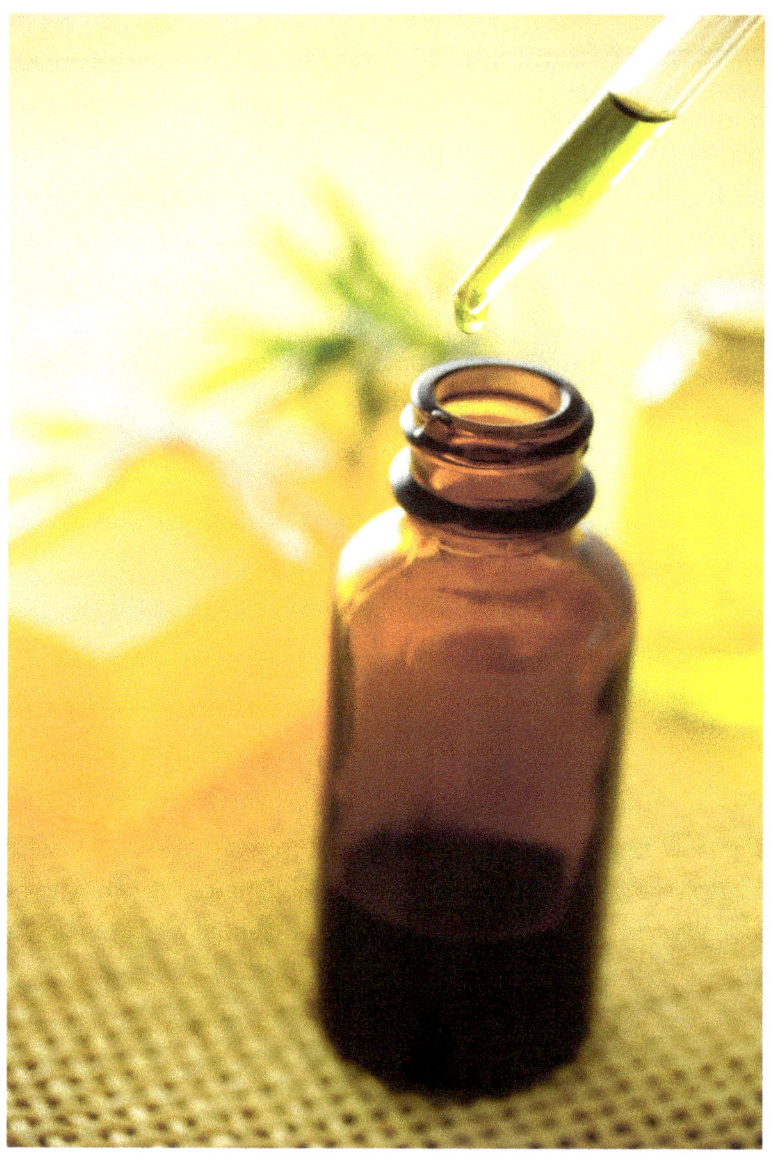

Hair Restoration, Enhancing Peppermint Oil

It helps to understand the chemistry of essential oils and the hair to appreciate the benefits they give. For example, peppermint oil, though not as versatile a treatment as other hair care focused blends; it is an all-important formula. As a homemade hair treatment, it restores balance to the hair network. Its primary role is to stimulate and control a healthy flow of blood to the roots of the hair. The process is essential as it gives the right amount of nourishment to all areas, including the scalp and follicles. In fact, regrowth and repair are unlikely to happen if this systematized process lacks efficiency.

The above mentioned essential oils are the primary ones to use as safe hair treatment solutions. Other variants of Essential oils can give acceptable results, but these are extremely favorable which, is credit to their reputation as natural hair remedies. Fragrant oils such as Rosemary and Lavender works effectively with variants of carrier oils to enhance their potency level. Additionally, combining different essential oils is a forward-thinking way to reach optimal satisfaction. Honestly speaking, it depends on the result the user intends to achieve.

The term carrier oils describe the function because these serve as transport agents for essential oils. Usually they are vegetable or oil-based stimulants extracted from nuts or seeds. In an unadulterated form, carrier oils are at extreme potency levels to preserve Essential oils. The two main processes used to extract the essence of carrier oils are maceration and cold pressing. As hair treatment boosters, carrier oils give the scalp a vast amount of moisture. This is to keep it well-nourished as it strengthens the tresses. Some commonly used variants of carrier oils include; Castor oil, Olive oil, Vitamin E oil, Avocado oil, Jojoba oil and coconut oil.

Few people acknowledge this fact, but the hair reflects how healthy and content a person is with their being. Additionally, it helps to boost self-confidence as a person cultivates a sense of integrity that represents his or her self-image. Essential oils and carrier emollients are all-natural, inexpensive hair treatment solutions. This makes achieving a healthy, voluminous network of tresses doable and manageable. It makes sense to exercise some basic precautionary steps when deciding to take a natural approach to hair care. This includes factoring aspects such as hair type when using essential oils as treatments.

About the Author

Amy Zulpa has quite a number of interests and essential oil is something that she has been interested in ever since her friend Melissa introduced her to the oils and the benefits that came with using them. From the personal experience that she has had using essential oils, she has made it her point of duty to spread the word on the benefits of the oils.

As Amy is also aware of the fact that many persons are seeking alternate methods to deal with minor ailments and for general health and wellness, her decision to write a book is well timed.

www.ingramcontent.com/pod-product-compliance
Ingram Content Group UK Ltd.
Pitfield, Milton Keynes, MK11 3LW, UK
UKHW021828270726
14058UKWH00001B/43

9 781680 323917